MUST HAVE

HOW TO CRUSH MEDICAL SCHOOL

TIPS ON HOW TO ACE YOUR MEDICAL SCHOOL CARRIER

DR. BILLY PONT

Copyright © 2022
Dr. Billy Pont
All rights reserved

DEDICATION

I dedicated this book to Medical personnel, teachers and students out there. You guys are AMAZING!

TABLE OF CONTENTS

INTRODUCTION 2

CHAPTER 1 6
SOME FACTS ABOUT MEDICAL SCHOOL YOU SHOULD KNOW 6

CHAPTER 2 14
FIRST YEAR IN MEDICAL SCHOOL 14

CHAPTER 3 18
HOW TO STUDY IN MEDICAL SCHOOL EFFECTIVELY 18

CHAPTER 4 24
CUT YOUR STUDY TIME INTO HALF 24

CHAPTER 5 26
HOW TO MANAGE MONEY IN MEDICAL SCHOOL 26

INTRODUCTION

Being a medical student will likely require you to work harder than you have ever worked before, but it will also likely require you to have more fun than you have ever had before. Many people use the fire hydrant analogy for medical school, but in reality, being a medical student is enjoyable, interesting, and extremely rewarding. There are a lot of off-putting myths about it.

Medical school is comparable to eating full pancakes every day. Doesn't that sound great? Who isn't a fan of pancakes?

However, there is a catch: anything you don't eat today will show up tomorrow. You'll feel sick and overwhelmed if you don't plan your "eating" ahead of time. Every day, there are pancakes on a plate.

Individually, it isn't difficult, the classes in medical school are similar to those in colleges in terms of difficulty, the ability to remain consistent is the most difficult aspect of medical school.

See, medical school is not as difficult as it seems. However, presenting medical school as a contest of willpower rather than intelligence is just not as entertaining. Therefore, medical school is portrayed as a terrifying environment.

You can learn how to do well in medical school without having to deal with too much stress if you follow the advice and strategies in this book.

As medical students, we are all aware of the vastness of our fields and the innumerable syndromes, clinical conditions, and drugs we must memorize. None of this can be accomplished by studying alone because the ratio of material to time is almost 50:1.

I worked tirelessly and was unsuccessful, i found out ways to improve my approach and discovered some methods for crushing medical school. I outlined how to learn and the qualities an ideal learner should have.

I figured out some fundamental learning skills that will help students even after completing medical school, i described some strategies on how to survive medical school based on my own experiences.

I am someone who is a visual learner and have a hard time understanding by simply reading the text. Once I am unable to visualize the information, it is difficult for me to remember it. This is not the case for everyone because each person has a different way of comprehending information, i accurately and precisely broke down each aspect of medical school as well as concepts and devised strategies that are not at all difficult to adapt in this book.

All that is required of you is motivation to follow. Additionally, i discussed the significance of discipline and time management in the medical field. I, like the majority of the other medical students, struggle to strike a balance between studying and socializing as a medical student. We frequently hold the belief that studying all day is necessary for success and necessitates sacrificing friends, family, and so on.

with this book, you can fulfill your wishes of doing well in medical school, pass all of your tests, and study like a pro.

After you finish reading this, you will learn how you can unfairly advantage yourself in medical school!

CHAPTER 1

SOME FACTS ABOUT MEDICAL SCHOOL YOU SHOULD KNOW

Being a medical student will likely require you to work harder than you have ever worked before, but you will also likely have more fun than you have ever had before. There are a lot of unsettling myths about being a medical student, but in reality, it is fun, interesting, and very rewarding, especially when you consider what you are pursuing.

Below are some facts you should know about medical school;

1. **What you learn can be put to good use for the rest of your life;** Despite the fact that it may appear to be a minor detail, it should not be ignored. Most of the time, all you really are studying for is to pass exams, and once you do that, the information you worked so hard to learn is mostly pointless. In medicine, subjects like anatomy, physiology, biochemistry, pharmacology, and pathology can all be used to diagnose, comprehend, and treat a disease. This is absolutely not the case. In addition to being a great incentive to learn the core course material well so that you will be a competent

doctor, this is also a great incentive to go beyond the basic lecture material and satisfy your curiosity about what you have been taught. A doctor might one day use this additional information in a clinical setting, and it could make a big difference for a patient. You don't just study for the next test when you study medicine, In addition, you are beginning a journey of lifelong learning that will lay the groundwork for your professional knowledge throughout your career in medicine.

2. **There is more to being a medical student than just studying medicine**; The things you can do in your spare time aren't just for having fun. Even though you do them for fun and to distract yourself from work, they are very important to your personal development. As previously stated, this involves working on skills that aren't covered in school but are still essential to being a good doctor. Because medicine is a career, it is essential to graduate from college as a functioning individual who is able to communicate effectively with others. This cannot be accomplished by studying the lecture notes every night in your room, it is essential to strike a healthy balance between work and life.

3. **While studying medicine, you will meet some of your closest friends**; Take advantage of the people with whom you are studying at university to the fullest. They need not necessarily be medical professionals; While many people form close

friendships with members of their sports team or society, it appears that medical professionals stick around together. Unfortunately, this can occasionally result in somewhat geeky "medic chat," in which, before you know what's going on, you start talking about the morning's lectures or how you found the practical the week before. This can help you remember what happened earlier in the lecture.

4. **Medical school keeps you up to date on the most recent medical research;** The study of medicine is a fantastic opportunity for those who have a genuine interest in the biological sciences to be brought very close to the frontier of current scientific knowledge, beyond what you will find in textbooks. Your professors are all actively involved in their respective fields, so it is their responsibility to keep abreast of the most recent research and developments. As a result, they are able to instruct subjects long before they appear in textbooks and introduce you to cutting-edge and pertinent research papers.

5. **Anatomy is more than just looking at pictures;** The first year of anatomy can be quite intense, as you dissect a "subject" who has chosen to donate their body to medical students in training. This means using a scalpel yourself and performing a task that can sometimes be quite unpleasant. Some people might be really excited about the idea of getting

started on a really hands-on anatomy course, but those who don't should not worry.
6. **The key is organization;** Learning at college is a genuine difference to being an understudy at school and one of the genuine difficulties is coordinating your work and exercises. You now have to organize things on your own rather than relying on your parents to keep track of everything. The combination of excessive studying or partying and the fact that most of your time at university will be spent exhausted is a recipe for disaster. Rehearsals and tutorials may conflict, and practical may coincide with sporting events. The most important thing is to have a system, whether it's a calendar on your phone or a paper diary you keep with you. Make sure you're not the one who always runs around trying to figure out where you're supposed to be or nearly misses something.
7. **The majority of your peers will be very smart;** Medical students are a very small group of people your age, and they will typically be very skilled and dedicated. When you compare yourself to other doctors, this can sometimes make you feel pretty down, especially since you'll usually notice the ones working harder than you are. Keep in mind that the people to whom you are comparing yourself are the very best students in the nation, so you shouldn't be discouraged if some of them are better than you. In fact, there will be many other

medical students at your level who are making the most of their education to grow as people and not just as students.

8. **Medicine takes time;** Medical school is more like a marathon than a sprint. It is a course that lasts five or six years, during which time you take fewer vacations and study almost all year (instead of just three months a year). The amount of information that needs to be learned is the reason the course is so long; teaching must cover both the fundamentals of science and the clinical skills needed to put them into practice. While this may appear to be an enormous undertaking, the reality is that time seems to fly by incredibly quickly at university. This is probably due to the fact that the average student is so busy that they do not have time to notice how quickly each term goes by. While this is nice because it makes you feel like you're moving quickly through your studies, it also means that it's easy to fall behind on work and won't catch up until after the holidays. Because of the short length of the terms, you can usually get away with this, and the holidays are often a good time to review the work from the previous term before the chaos of term time starts all over again.

9. **Not everything is hard work;** Don't worry, medicine can be hard, but you'll still have plenty of time to enjoy your time as an undergraduate, which many people consider to be the best time of their lives.

You will have time to take advantage of other university activities like sports, music, and the vast array of other societies that are available to you because of the course's level of work. Be effective with the time you spend working in order to manage these additional activities, if you know you have a music rehearsal that evening, don't waste an entire afternoon watching videos on YouTube. You will learn a lot about yourself and other people while attending university, and you will hopefully develop into someone who is capable of being a good doctor. However, attending university is about much more than just earning a degree.

10. **You will become a doctor if you pass your exams;** If you pass all of your exams while studying medicine, you will eventually become a doctor, barring any catastrophe. Although it may appear obvious, it is worth taking a step back and considering this. A university certifies that you are competent enough to continue your education toward becoming a doctor by granting you a passing score on an exam. How does this affect you? First of all, it indicates that passing exams can be challenging. In other subjects, you are considered competent if you get a good grade (typically a 2:1), but if you pass medicine, you are guaranteed to go on to clinical school and a professional medical career. Even though passing exams can be particularly challenging, this is also a very exciting

prospect. You will be qualified as a doctor if you are able to continue at a reasonable level and put in enough effort. If things get tough and you think you might have trouble passing, keep in mind that passing is one step closer to becoming a doctor.

CHAPTER 2

FIRST YEAR IN MEDICAL SCHOOL

You've been accepted to medical school!
Congrats! But now, which errors should medical students in their first year absolutely avoid?
It was terrible when I started medical school! I had no idea how to study in this unfamiliar setting. I considered altering my behavior because I was feeling so defeated.
I was being urged to study harder by everyone. It was the most difficult time of my life because I had to make a change, even though I had studied the most.
I looked for the problem for months. I discovered these strategies that should not be ignored by medical students, I was studying hard enough, but I wasn't studying in the right way that was the problem!
As a medical student, I became the best version of myself, the results of this work were incredible even though I was studying less than before, I had better grades, which was impressive.
I was able to pass all of my tests and still have time for my hobbies, friends, and other interests, that's when I realized I was not to blame, all these years of failure were actually caused by the fact that school has always only told us to study hard.

Some tips for your first days at med school; -
1. **Don't arrive with a preconceived notion:**
   Please don't be the student who comes in and says they only want to study and want to become a dermatologist, orthopedic surgeon, or plastic surgeon.

   Yes, you will need to put in a lot of effort to achieve these fantastic goals. But don't let them stop you from having a good time in medical school.

   You don't have to give up your sanity to become the specialist of your dreams. I am aware of students who are not only the smartest but also the most well-rounded.

2. **Avoid Using Passive Strategies Too Much:**
   One of these students was me. I spent between 60 and 80 percent of my time using passive methods like reading the material, taking notes, and watching the lecture, then I would put myself to the test in the remaining time.

   I quickly realized that this 60/40 split was not going to work because I am a typical test taker.

   As a result, I was able to devise a study strategy that satisfied me. I reduced my passive methods from 60% to 30%. Because of that, I was able to complete flashcards and practice questions for the majority of my time.

   What took place with my grade? They exploded!
   What became of my spare time? also shot up a lot!

I was frequently asked, "Was I even in medical school? When that happens, you know you've found a method that works.

3. **Plan medical school around your life, not your life around medical school:**

   When you make this change, there are two outcomes.

   First, your interests are still present in your life.

   Second, when you study, you force yourself to become more efficient. You have deliberately scheduled less time, so you can no longer waste it.

   As a result, you get rid of the useless material that hurts your retention and final grade.

   The end result is a medical student in their first year who manages to balance their passions with their studies.

4. **Get Patient Exposure Right Away:**

   We are going to medical school to become doctors, but our first year of school is not particularly busy. That doesn't make sense.

   Although a lot of schools are updating their curricula, many institutions still restrict the amount of patient exposure their first-year medical students receive.

   It could be a form of cuddling and holding hands. However, you should make every effort to see as many patients as possible as soon as possible.

   While it is essential to understand the human body's anatomy, physiology, and pathology, you will probably retain the most information through hands-on experience.

Therefore, look for patient exposure in your city, such as free clinics. You can give back to your community by volunteering at health-related events like health fairs and blood banks.

These experiences will motivate you to continue attending medical school, but the most important benefit of this early exposure is that it will help you get past the difficult learning curve that comes with providing excellent patient care. There is frequently a phase of awkwardness because you are not used to talking to patients.

Therefore, get started right away and start acting like a doctor! You'll be glad you did that in your third and fourth years.

CHAPTER 3

HOW TO STUDY IN MEDICAL SCHOOL EFFECTIVELY

How can we actively study in medical school and study less? What are the strategies for studying less and getting better grades?

In reality, different methods of studying for medical school will work for different people, but a single person may employ multiple methods. You must determine which approaches will provide you with the best outcomes in the shortest amount of time.

In medical school, you'll hear a lot about active versus passive learning. If you haven't heard of it, passive studying involves doing things like reading the syllabus, looking at the slides, copying your notes exactly, and so on.

Practice questions, flashcards, asking questions, and explaining concepts to your peers are all examples of active learning.

Although it may appear obvious which approach should be taken during medical school, the majority of students spend the majority of their time passively learning. You can use each of the below methods actively or passively.

1. **Using Flashcards**

Utilizing flashcards has made the difference between studying efficiently and wasting countless hours in medical school.

Active is using flashcards. However, students frequently make the mistake of making too many cards and not having enough time to review them all. Your flashcards ought to be about subjects with high yields. For instance, if you are learning about a disease, the disease's mechanism, symptoms, diagnosis, and treatment should be covered on the flashcards.

You should give them a try in classes like microbiology, anatomy, and pharmacology.

2. **Using Your Syllabus**

The majority of students will prepare for the lecture by reading the syllabus beforehand. This could be as simple as highlighting relevant information. Taking notes on the side is another possibility.

It's fine if you highlight to familiarize yourself with the lecture. However, this should not take more than 15 to 20 minutes for each lecture. If so, you may as well be actively reading because you are reading too thoroughly.

Knowing the lecture topic, writing down some straightforward questions about it, skimming the material, and then responding to as many of your questions as you can is a great way to make pre-reading active. After pre-reading, you may have general responses to some of these questions but have no idea about others. After class, you should pay attention to questions you don't understand and think more deeply about questions you do understand.

You can't go wrong with using the syllabus as your primary resource because important information and exam questions frequently come from it.

Ensure that the method you choose is as active and effective as possible. You will work fewer hours as a result of this.

3. **Using Outlines**

    Using outlines as a method of study is another common practice in medical school.

    Condense your notes from the lecture and syllabus into a Word document or sheet of paper. You can also annotate the notes next to each slide with a program like OneNote.

    It is an excellent method for condensing lecture material. Just be careful not to spend too much time creating the outlines and too little time actually studying them. Concentrate on the lecture and syllabus points with the highest yield. First, learn these, then return to the specifics.

    If you succeed, you might be able to study for a test using 20 to 30 pages from your outline instead of more than 500 pages from your syllabus.

4. **Group Studying**

During your four years in medical school, your classmates will be some of your most valuable resources. Form a study group with people who share your interests and are equally or more intelligent than you.

I believe that group study should only be used if you are familiar with the material. Don't expect to learn everything when you join your group studying. You need to devise a structure for your group's learning and accountability practices.

Therefore, schedule a time to meet with your peers and discuss your concerns. You might be able to use questions that you made with your flashcards or that you annotated on your slides.

Be attentive during the study group because your group members may be more knowledgeable than you about a question. The most important thing is to decide what you will cover and how much time you will spend studying that day. Make sure you have a strategy and come prepared.

5. **Using Active Listening**

Believe it or not, there are students who are able to attend a lecture for three hours without writing or typing anything down. Although they are smart, as are all of us, they have determined that they are auditory learners and must therefore actively listen. If this describes you, you should set yourself the challenge of asking the lecturer one or two questions. If you're too worried about coming across as "that one guy" in class, you can do this during lecture, via email, or even after class. Always make sure to ask questions!

6. **Be Sure to Exercise**

    Exercise has many physical and mental benefits, which are especially important for stressed-out medical school students. You should incorporate regular exercise into your day to relieve stress and lower your anxiety levels. Try stair runs, wall sits, chair dips, mountain climbers, or an at-home exercise app if getting to the gym is difficult.

7. **Reward Yourself**

    Getting through medical school can be difficult and mentally and physically taxing. When you reach your goals, it's important to reward yourself. These rewards need not be extravagant or costly; rather, they should just make you feel better and serve as a special treat as you move closer to achieving your objectives.

CHAPTER 4

CUT YOUR STUDY TIME INTO HALF

Have you ever avoided watching Dr. Najeeb video lectures because they were too long? What if I told you that you could use speed listening in medical school and cut your studying time in half?
speed-listening is something that should be tried by every medical student. Perhaps you are not yet convinced. You might argue that it is already difficult enough to listen to your lectures at 1x, much less 2x. I don't know about you, but I wouldn't sit through a lecture for an hour and only remember 18 minutes. If you take into account how simple it is to switch from not paying attention to paying attention, this number is probably even lower.
When you can use it in just 1.5 hours, why spend three? Consider whether you'd rather attend lectures five days a week or two and a half days a week.
You can extend your study time by using speed listening if you assume that you have four one-and-a-half-hour lectures each day throughout the course of the week.
In medical school, we do not want to spend three hours a day on a passive method.
Instead, in medical school, speed listening can help you cut down on your study time by half or more.

So, how can you speed up your videos so that you can stream lectures faster in medical school?

1) **The free Chrome extension Video Speed Controller:**
   With Video Speed Controller, you can speed up any video by up to four times. After downloading the free tool, you can simply use your keyboard to speed up or slow down videos.

   This is applicable to any HTML5 file, which is practically every video we watch. As a result, Video Speed Controller can speed through school training modules or YouTube videos!

2) **Using VLC Player:**
   Despite the fact that the Video Speed Controller is an excellent tool for watching videos online, what program do you use to watch videos on your desktop?

   The free media player VLC lets you speed up videos up to 16 times. Naturally, you won't need to repeat 2-3 times.

3) **Using Audipo to Quickly Listen on Your Mobile Device:**

CHAPTER 5

HOW TO MANAGE MONEY IN MEDICAL SCHOOL

As a medical student, sticking to a budget is a crucial step in reducing the amount of debt you will have to pay back. Try to approach a budget in the same way that you would a healthy diet. You will benefit from making responsible decisions that are sensible.

Smart budgeting is one of the best ways to keep your finances in check while you study to be a doctor.

Below are some tips on how you can manage your expenses at medical school

1. **Cook with your classmates:**

    You can either cook several portions at a time to freeze for the week or join a cooking co-op with other students. Not only is participating in a cooking cooperative a more social way to spend mealtime, but it also saves time overall when cooking. You can even quiz each other on the materials from the class. It's also a great chance to learn some new recipes and meal plans from your classmates and friends. Additionally, purchasing groceries in bulk may be less expensive than purchasing individual portions.

2. **Keep track of your spending:**

To get a complete picture of where your money is actually going, try keeping every receipt for a few months. You can use this information to figure out where you might need to cut back.

3. **Do not quickly buy brand new medical books or equipment:**

   At the end of their time in medical school, upperclassmen almost always are willing to sell things. You can buy, sell, or even swap books on a lot of websites. If you and your friends require the same books or a number of titles, you might be able to qualify for free shipping by purchasing your purchases together, which will save you a lot of money.

4. **Set a monthly allowance**

   Having a goal can be helpful. Based on the anticipated costs for the school year, determine a monthly budget. Try to stay within your monthly limit, even when making credit-based purchases. You can always adjust to reflect reality, even if you don't get it right every month.

5. **Shop Smart**

   You might save time by buying groceries online. Always bring a list with you when you go shopping to cut down on impulsive purchases and time spent browsing.

   Utilize manufacturer coupons while planning your menu around weekly sales.

   Never buy unnecessarily things

6. **Start educating yourself in finances early**

   You cannot expect to learn the fundamentals of finance from your residency or medical school. Worst of all, a lot of "salesmen" will take advantage of this just as you start making money. Make decisions about your financial future!

www.ingramcontent.com/pod-product-compliance
Lightning Source LLC
Chambersburg PA
CBHW050325220526
45465CB00005B/2133